AF444526

Contents

What exactly is sex? 3

What is Desire? 8

   Formation of Desire 10

   The Scent of Attraction 14

   A Potent Cocktail...17

   Mysteries of Desire 22

Sexual Desire...24

   Differences Between Sexual Arousal and Desire 26

Sex Drive: How Do Men and Women Compare?..........33

   9 Ways For Men to Improve Sexual Performance 47

   9 Safe Ways to Increase Female Libido.................55

What are sex pills? 67

   What are the best sex pills available?...................68

   What are erection pills?.......................................70

   Are male enhancement pills dangerous? 72

   Are there sex pills for women? 75

   Other things you can do to improve the sex you're having...80

Factors affecting sexual desire...................................82

What exactly is sex?

Society typically tells us that there are two sexes: male and female. You may also be familiar with the fact that some people are intersex, or have a difference of sexual development (DSD).

DSD is used to describe chromosomes, anatomy, or sex characteristics that can't be categorized as exclusively male or female.

As with names and pronouns, it's important to refer to people in the manner that they prefer. Some people are comfortable with the term "intersex" and use it to describe themselves. Others have moved away from using this term and refer to their condition as a DSD.

With some research reporting that as many as 1 in 100Trusted Source people are born with a DSD, more biologistsTrusted Source are acknowledging that sex may be far more complex than what the traditional male-female binary accounts for.

Genitalia

Some believe genitals determine sex, with males having penises and females having vaginas.

However, this definition excludes some people with a DSD.

It can also invalidate trans people who are non-operative — those who don't want to have bottom surgery — or pre-operative.

For example, a transgender man — a person who was assigned female at birth and identifies as a man — may have a vagina but still identify as male.

Chromosomes

We're typically taught that people with XX chromosomes are female and people with XY chromosomes are male.

This excludes folks with a DSD who may have different chromosomal configurations or other differences in sexual development.

It also doesn't account for the fact that trans people often have chromosomes that don't "match" their sex. A transgender woman, for example, can be female but still have XY chromosomes.

Primary sex characteristics

We tend to associate a predominance of estrogen with females and a predominance of testosterone with males. It's important to understand that every person has both of these hormones.

In fact, estradiol, the predominant form of estrogen, is critical to sexual functionTrusted Source for people who were assigned male at birth. Estradiol plays a significant role in sexual arousal, sperm production, and erectile function.

Although hormone replacement therapy is an option for trans and gender non-conforming people, a trans man who isn't on hormones, for example, isn't any less male than one who is.

Secondary sex characteristics

Many secondary sex characteristics are easily identifiable. This includes facial hair, breast tissue, and vocal range.

Because of this, they're often used to make quick assessments about sex.

But secondary sex characteristics vary greatly, regardless of whether someone identifies with the sex they were assigned at birth.

Take facial hair, for example. Some people who were assigned female at birth may go on to develop facial hair, and some who were assigned male at birth may not grow any at all.

What is Desire?

Typically, we tend to think of desire as an emotion — that is, arising from our mental status, akin to affection or anger or grief or surprise or ecstasy. But this is probably not the case. Many scientists and psychologists now believe that desire is, in fact, a bodily urge, more analogous to hunger or the blood's need for oxygen. For anyone who has been maddeningly in love, driven to the edge of despair by an unquenchable desire for another, this probably doesn't seem so far-fetched. In many ways we can't control what we desire because it is a hard-wired emotional and physiological response."

 No surprise: desire and sexuality are practically inextricable. The word "desire" probably brings to mind tawny romance novels, adult-only activities, and a longing for sexual connection. Sexual desire may in fact be the only type of desire; psychoanalytic theory holds that all other forms of desire and creative energy are the result of rerouted sexual energy — often called "the libido" — towards other endeavors. The bodily urge of desire is only sexual in nature; everything else is an emotional state developed out of this primary desire.

Whether or not you buy that, it is clear that sexual desire is one of the — if not the — strongest of human needs. Typically, it takes up a huge portion of our time, emotional energy, and lives. Why? What drives the often unstoppable freight train of sexual desire?

Formation of Desire

Desire is the coming together of visual, biochemical, emotional, and biomechanical cues that trigger a hormonal cascade that may culminate in the successful fertilization of an egg by a sperm." A pretty clinical explanation, but one held widely throughout the profession and related fields of study. in essence, instincts rule our desire; the preferences we have in our sexual lives are, more or less, simply an expression of our search for evolutionary advantage.

A number of tenets of popular wisdom regarding sexual preference through an evolutionary appeal:

• Good looks are more important to men than they are to women because good looks

signal good health and thus an enhanced
ability to reproduce.

• Women find social standing essential in a
mate because that signals a capability to care
and protect their future children.

• Women prefer older men because they are
more likely to have the resources to provide
for them and their children.

Buss claims that these and a few other basic
instincts drive desire and are the same across
all cultures and societies. When it comes
down to it, for Buss and many others, it's all
about the need to reproduce.

Obviously, Buss's explanation greatly
simplifies the complexity of human
sexuality. Some might argue that he
simplifies it to the point of offense. Where,
for example, do men who prefer men as

sexual partners fit into this explanation? Or women who prefer women? And why do people who are physically unable to reproduce still feel sexual desire? Nevertheless, the argument is compelling.

Desire is indeed based on an evolutionary need," he said. "We have a very strong, sometimes unconscious desire to perpetuate our species. The expression of sexual desire — our conscious feelings and our performances of sexuality — is far more complex than just trying to have babies.

The expression of sexual desire is most likely rooted in childhood. As stress-management expert Debbie Mandel points out, "children observe their parents and absorb lessons about parental sexuality and desire." Although at first we do not have the

ability or the occasion to express them, these
initial impressions of desire are not lost on
us. When we enter puberty, we start to feel
the evolutionary desire towards
reproduction. Immediately, this desire
begins to express itself as the learned
sexuality we have been soaking up since
childhood. As we grow older, it changes as
it is shaped by social cues from our peers
and by mass media portrayals. It may take
one of any number of forms; though desire
may be simple, sexuality is multifarious and
varied. Sexuality is the expression of desire,
and the aspect of desire we can access,
manipulate, and enjoy.

The Scent of Attraction

Sexual desire itself is a drive lodged deep in the gut, working without our knowledge and beyond our control. we are attracted to one another on a subconscious level, as the result of biomechanical cues, including posture and the pheromones they give off — their sexual "scent" — that cause us to choose the mates we do. Perfume manufacturers and ad-men have latched onto this theory of pheromones, marketing scents that supposedly will "help you attract sexual attention instantly from the opposite sex!" But what are they actually selling?

Pheromones are chemical signals sent out by one member of a species in order to trigger a natural response in another member of that same species. It's been well observed that pheromones are used by animals, especially insects, to communicate with each other on sublingual levels. The menstrual cycles of women who live together in close quarters tend to become synchronized over time. This effect is caused by human female pheromone communication and that this is only one example of a type of sexual communication that is constantly occurring between humans on the sublingual level.

talk to the sex centers of the brain and can trigger a release of specific sex hormones," testosterone and estrogen. The effects of pheromones are clearest in cases where, for example "couples who for every reason should be disinterested in each other suddenly can't stay out of each other's presence after an 'up-close-and-personal encounter'" — coworkers on a business trip, for example.

In recent years, scientists have begun to suspect that a little-known cranial nerve may be the key to the mysterious workings of pheromones. First discovered in humans in 1913, the "cranial nerve zero" or "terminal nerve" runs from the nasal cavity to the brain, ending in what Dr. Fields calls "the hot-button sex regions of the brain." For years, scientists believed that nerve zero was part of the olfactory nerve, helping our brain interpret smells.The brain of a pilot whale had no olfactory nerve whatsoever, it did have nerve zero. What difference does a whale brain make? Whales long ago evolved to lose the ability to smell, their noses becoming blowholes. And yet, though whales no longer have neural hardware for smell, they still have nerve zero, connecting the whale's blowhole to its brain and other experiments, discovering that stimulating nerve zero triggered automatic sexual responses in animals.

Scholars believe that cranial nerve zero may be responsible for translating the signals of sex pheromones and initiating reproductive behavior. In other words, cranial nerve zero may be the bio-machinery for desire.

A Potent Cocktail

Pheromones may act as a kind of stoplight for sexual desire. They let us know that we're good to go, but they certainly don't work alone. Regardless what turned it on, something's still got to be driving the car. It turns out to be an intoxicating mix of hormones and neurochemicals firing in the brain.That "hot-button sex region" is the septal nucleus, which, among other things, controls the release of the two primary sex hormones in the body: testosterone and estrogen. Both hormones are essential in the process of desire. Scientists know this, because as men grow older, they tend to lose testosterone and, as a result, develop erection and libido problems. Women also lose testosterone as they age. However, due to poor results from tests involving testosterone administration in women with a loss of sexual desire, scientists now believe that a combination of testosterone and estrogen is the ultimate "love hormone."

Estrogen and testosterone, in turn, stimulate neurochemicals in the brain — specifically, dopamine, serotonin, norapenephine and oxytocin. The combination of neurochemicals triggers dizzying feelings of excitement, euphoria, and passion," he said. "Some brain imaging studies show a similarity between neural activity in subjects with obsessive-compulsive disorder and those who are falling in love." Love — or at least desire — literally drives you crazy. How? What are these chemicals actually doing?

• Dopamine - Dopamine has mostly been studied in the context of drug addiction. Essentially, it's the neurotransmitter that makes external stimuli arousing. Dopamine trains you to associate the feeling of being satiated and pleasured with certain things. In the case of sexual desire, dopamine is released in the brain whenever you encounter something to which or someone to whom you're attracted.

• Serotonin - Serotonin is similar to dopamine; it is a neurotransmitter that teaches your body a cycle of desire and satisfaction.

• Norapenephrine - Usually, this neurotransmitter is stimulated when we need extra energy to escape a dangerous or scary situation. But it also tends to increase during masturbation and sex, peaking at orgasm and then declining.

• Oxytocin Oxytocin has been called the "cuddle hormone." It is believed to play an essential role in parent-child bonding and in partner formation. A 1992 study by the National Institute of Mental Health of the prairie vole — an animal known for being firmly monogamous — showed that when forming a bond with a mate, the vole's brain releases a rush of oxytocin. Even more telling, when oxytocin is blocked, the vole can't make a connection at all. Oxytocin doesn't cause arousal, but it may be part of the overall drive that is desire. According to Dr. Malkin, it "relaxes our guard and deepens trust."

Various studies through the years have shown that all of these neurochemicals and more (including epinephrine, alpha melanocyte polypeptide, phenethylamine, and gonadotropins), are in one way or another involved in sexual desire. But when it comes down to it, it's pretty much impossible to isolate any one mechanism. It's helpful to take a small step back to see why.

Mysteries of Desire

When the technology to look at brain activity during sexual stimulation became available, scientists expected it to show a fairly straight path from visual recognition to emotional/sexual interest. And yet the brain-imaging showed that sexual desire creates an incredibly intricate and non-linear network of brain activity, including lighting up regions in the brain typically devoted to "higher" functions, such as self-awareness and understanding others, prior to lighting up the more straightforward physical-response sections. It all happens incredibly fast and often below the radar of consciousness. In many cases, people do not even seem to know what turns them on.

The interaction of neurochemicals involved in desire is dense and convoluted. And the mechanics of what may turn out to be the most essential element of desire - phermones and cranial nerve zero - still remains unclear. All of this confusion does help to explain why treatment methods for loss of libido seem at best haphazard and often ineffective. In many cases, placebos tend to work just as well as the real thing. [If you're interested, yes, Viagra works, but it doesn't actually affect desire; it affects arousal, an entirely different bodily mechanism (and a whole other discussion)].

Maybe the confusion isn't so bad. What's nice about the inability of science to fully unravel this mystery is that it keeps some of the magic of love and desire alive. After all, if desire was a thing known, perhaps it would no longer be a thing to keep us going.

Sexual Desire

Is a motivational state and an interest in "sexual objects or activities, or as a wish, or drive to seek out sexual objects or to engage in sexual activities". Synonyms for sexual desire are libido, sexual attraction and lust. Sexual desire is an aspect of a person's sexuality, which varies significantly from one person to another, and also varies depending on circumstances at a particular time. Not every person experiences sexual desire; those who do not experience it may be labeled asexual.

Sexual desire may be the "single most common sexual event in the lives of men and women". Sexual desire is a subjective feeling state that can "be triggered by both internal and external cues, and that may or may not result in overt sexual behavior". Sexual desire can be aroused through imagination and sexual fantasies, or perceiving an individual whom one finds attractive. Sexual desire is also created and amplified through sexual tension, which is caused by sexual desire that has yet to be consummated.

Sexual desire can be spontaneous or responsive. Sexual desire is dynamic, can either be positive or negative, and can vary in intensity depending on the desired object/person. The sexual desire spectrum are: aversion → disinclination → indifference → interest → need → passion.

The production and use of sexual fantasy and thought is an important part of properly functioning sexual desire. Some physical manifestations of sexual desire in humans are; licking, sucking, puckering and touching the lips, as well as tongue protrusion.

Differences Between Sexual Arousal and Desire

It's easy to conflate libido with arousal. After all, if you feel satisfied with your sex life, these aspects of your sexuality can be difficult to separate from one another. In actuality, libido refers to your baseline interest in sex, and may also be referred to as your sexual appetite or desire.

Arousal, on the other hand, refers to your physiological response to sexual stimuli. Physical manifestations of sexual arousal include vaginal lubrication and increased blood flow to the labia, clitoris, and vagina.

Sexual desires in women tend to fluctuate throughout their lifetimes, and there are many different causative factors. Basically, low sexual desire (HSDD) and the inability to experience or maintain sexual arousal (sexual arousal disorder) are quite common. Studies say that nearly half of all women experience at least one symptom of sexual dysfunction at some point.1

An Overview of Hypoactive Sexual Desire Disorder

Difficulties with Sexual Desire and Arousal

The current diagnostic and statistical manual of mental disorder, the Diagnostic and Statistical Manual of Mental Disorders (DSM–5), classifies problems with arousal and desire together, under the term Female Sexual Interest/Arousal Disorders (FSAID).2

Women with FSAID may experience a decrease in their desire for sex and may not initiate sex or be responsive to initiation attempts. They may also notice that they are not easily (or even ever) aroused and that excitement or pleasure during sex is reduced.

A woman must meet three out of the six criteria set out by the DSM to receive a FSAID diagnosis—all of which revolve around one's interest and response to sexual activity.

Diagnostic Criteria for FSAID

• Absent or reduced interest in sexual activity

• Absent or reduced sexual thoughts or fantasies

• No or reduced initiation of sexual activity, and typically unreceptive to a partner's attempts to initiate

• Absent or reduced sexual excitement or pleasure in almost all or all sexual encounters

• Absent or reduced sexual interest/arousal in response to any internal or external sexual cues

• Absent or reduced genital or non-genital sensations during sexual activity in all or almost all sexual encounters

How to Increase Sexual Arousal Levels

One of the symptoms of decreased sexual arousal in women is a reduced amount of vaginal lubrication. Over-the-counter vaginal lubricants can augment lubrication.

If a decrease in vaginal lubrication has been caused by menopause, hormone replacement therapy is often prescribed. While this is an approved drug therapy for this problem, there are some risks and side effects that come with this treatment. For this reason, a personal lubricant purchased from your local pharmacy may be your safest option.

Choosing the Right Vaginal Lubricant for a Great Sex Life

Viagra (sildenafil) and a class of medications called alpha-adrenergic blockers, such as Regitine (phentolamine), have also been shown to increase vaginal lubrication in response to sexual stimulation. However, it should be mentioned that multiple studies on Viagra for various female sexual problems have not shown an increase in sexual pleasure in women, and it has still not been approved by the FDA for use with women.3

Aside from pharmacological solutions, you can also choose behavioral therapy to help increase sexual arousal. This therapy is aimed at enhancing sexual fantasies and focusing one's attention on sexual stimuli. If you are in an ongoing relationship, your therapist would also take a look at the possibility that communication problems exist in your relationship, or that your partner does not spend as much time as is needed to sexually stimulate you.

How to Increase Sexual Desire Levels

Addyi (flibanserin) is FDA-approved for the treatment of low sexual desire (HSDD). Addyi is a pill that must be taken every day and it's advisable to stay away from alcohol while on it because fainting can occur.4

Vyleesi, an injectable drug, has also been approved for the treatment of low sexual desire in pre-menopausal women. This drug is for women who previously had more satisfying levels of sexual desire but now experience low sexual desire. It is not for those whose low sexual desire is caused by other factors like an underlying medical condition or medication.5

There have also been studies indicating that testosterone can increase sexual desire in women whose low sex drive is a result of the surgical removal of their ovaries. Continual treatment with testosterone does, however, have side effects and health risks

Sex Drive: How Do Men and Women Compare?

Birds do it, bees do it, and men do it any old time. But women will only do it if the candles are scented just right -- and their partner has done the dishes first. A stereotype, sure, but is it true? Do men really have stronger sex drives than women?

Well, yes, they do. Study after study shows that men's sex drives are not only stronger than women's, but much more straightforward. The sources of women's libidos, by contrast, are much harder to pin down.

It's common wisdom that women place more value on emotional connection as a spark of sexual desire. But women also appear to be heavily influenced by social and cultural factors as well.

"Sexual desire in women is extremely sensitive to environment and context.

Here are seven patterns of men's and women's sex drives that researches have shown. Bear in mind that people may vary from these norms.

1. Men think more about sex.

The majority of adult men under 60 think about sex at least once a day. Only about one-quarter of women say they think about it that frequently. As men and women age, each fantasize less, but men still fantasize about twice as often.

In a survey of studies comparing male and female sex drives it is found that men reported more spontaneous sexual arousal and had more frequent and varied fantasies.

2. Men seek sex more avidly.

"Men want sex more often than women at the start of a relationship, in the middle of it, and after many years of it, after reviewing several surveys of men and women. This isn't just true of heterosexuals, he says; gay men also have sex more often than lesbians at all stages of the relationship. Men also say they want more sex partners in their lifetime, and are more interested in casual sex.

Men are more likely to seek sex even when it's frowned upon or even outlawed:

• About two-thirds say they masturbate, even though about half also say they feel guilty about it, Laumann says. By contrast, about 40% of women say they masturbate, and the frequency of masturbation is smaller among women.

• Prostitution is still mostly a phenomenon of men seeking sex with women, rather than the other way around.

• Nuns do a better job of fulfilling their vows of chastity than priests. A survey of several hundred clergy in which 62% of priests admitted to sexual activity, compared to 49% of nuns. The men reported more partners on average than the women.

3. Women's sexual turn-ons are more complicated than men's.

What turns women on? Not even women always seem to know. Northwestern University researcher Meredith Chivers and colleagues showed erotic films to gay and straight men and women. They asked them about their level of sexual arousal, and also measured their actual level of arousal through devices attached to their genitals.

For men, the results were predictable: Straight men said they were more turned on by depictions of male-female sex and female-female sex, and the measuring devices backed up their claims. Gay men said they were turned on by male-male sex, and again the devices backed them up. For women, the results were more surprising. Straight women, for example, said they were more turned on by male-female sex. But genitally they showed about the same reaction to male-female, male-male, and female-female sex.

"Men are very rigid and specific about who they become aroused by, who they want to have sex with, who they fall in love with. By contrast, women may be more open to same-sex relationships thanks to their less-directed sex drives, Bailey says. "Women probably have the capacity to become sexually interested in and fall in love with their own sex more than men do," "They won't necessarily do it, but they have the capacity."

The idea was backed up by studies showing that homosexuality is a more fluid state among women than men. In another broad review of studies, it is found many more lesbians reported recent sex with men, when compared to gay men's reports of sex with women. Women were also more likely than men to call themselves bisexual, and to report their sexual orientation as a matter of choice.

4. Women's sex drives are more influenced by social and cultural factors.

There are many ways in which women's sexual attitudes, practices, and desires were more influenced by their environment than men:

• Women's attitudes toward (and willingness to perform) various sexual practices are more likely than men's to change over time.

• Women who regularly attend church are less likely to have permissive attitudes about sex. Men do not show this connection between church attendance and sex attitudes.

• Women are more influenced by the attitudes of their peer group in their decisions about sex.

• Women with higher education levels were more likely to have performed a wider variety of sexual practices (such as oral sex); education made less of a difference with men.

• Women were more likely than men to show inconsistency between their expressed values about sexual activities such as premarital sex and their actual behavior.

• Why are women's sex drives seemingly weaker and more vulnerable to influence? Some have theorized it's related to the greater power of men in society, or differing sexual expectations of men when compared to women. Laumann prefers an explanation more closely tied to the world of sociobiology.

• Men have every incentive to have sex to pass along their genetic material, Laumann says. By contrast, women may be hard-wired to choose their partners carefully, because they are the ones who can get pregnant and wind up taking care of the baby. They are likely to be more attuned to relationship quality because they want a partner who will stay around to help take care of the child. They're also more likely to choose a man with resources because of his greater ability to support a child.

• 5. Women take a less direct route to sexual satisfaction.

•

• Men and women travel slightly different paths to arrive at sexual desire. "I hear women say in my office that desire originates much more between the ears than between the legs "For women there is a need for a plot -- hence the romance novel. It is more about the anticipation, how you get there; it is the longing that is the fuel for desire,"

• Women's desire "is more contextual, more subjective, more layered on a lattice of emotion," Men, by contrast, don't need to have nearly as much imagination, since sex is simpler and more straightforward for them.

• That doesn't mean men don't seek intimacy, love, and connection in a relationship, just as women do. They just view the role of sex differently. "Women want to talk first, connect first, then have sex," For men, sex is the connection. Sex is the language men use to express their tender loving vulnerable side," It is their language of intimacy.

• 6. Women experience orgasms differently than men.

• Men, on average, take 4 minutes from the point of entry until ejaculation. Women usually take around 10 to 11 minutes to reach orgasm -- if they do.

• That's another difference between the sexes: how often they have an orgasm during sex. Among men who are part of a couple, 75% say they always have an orgasm, as opposed to 26% of the women. And not only is there a difference in reality, there's one in perception, too. While the men's female partners reported their rate of orgasm accurately, the women's male partners said they believed their female partners had orgasms 45% of the time.

• 7. Women's libidos seem to be less responsive to drugs.

• With men's sex drives seemingly more directly tied to biology when compared to women, it may be no surprise that low desire may be more easily treated through medication in men. Men have embraced drugs as a cure not only for erectile dysfunction but also for a shrinking libido. With women, though, the search for a drug to boost sex drive has proved more elusive.

• Testosterone has been linked to sex drive in both men and women. But testosterone works much faster in men with low libidos than women. While the treatments are effective, they're not as effective in women as in men. "There is a hormonal factor in [sex drive], but it is much more important in men than women.

• A testosterone patch for women called Intrinsa has been approved in Europe but was rejected by the FDA due to concerns about long-term safety. But the drug has sparked a backlash from some medical and psychiatric professionals who question

whether low sex drive in women should
even be considered a condition best treated
with drugs. They point to the results of a
large survey in which about 40% of women
reported some sort of sexual problem --
most commonly low sexual desire -- but
only 12% said they felt distressed about it.
With all the factors that go into the stew that
piques sexual desire in women, some
doctors say a drug should be the last
ingredient to consider, rather than the first.

9 Ways For Men to Improve Sexual Performance

Improve male sexual performance

If you're looking to maintain sexual activity
in bed all night, you're not alone.

Many men are looking for ways to enhance their sexual performance. This can include improving existing problems or searching for new ways to keep your partner happy.

There are plenty of male enhancement pills on the market, but there are many simple ways to stay firmer and last longer without having to visit the pharmacy.

Keep in mind that your penis works on blood pressure, and make sure your circulatory system is working at top shape. Basically, what's good for your heart is good for your sexual health.

Keep reading to find other easy ways to improve your sexual performance.

1. Stay active

One of the best ways to improve your health is cardiovascular exercise. Sex might get your heart rate up, but regular exercise can help your sexual performance by keeping your heart in shape.

Thirty minutes a day of sweat-breaking exercise, such as running and swimming, can do wonders to boost your libido.

2. Eat these fruits and vegetables

Certain foods can also help you increase blood flow. They include:

• Onions and garlic. These foods may not be great for your breath, but they can help your blood circulation.

• Bananas. This potassium-rich fruit can help lower your blood pressure, which can benefit your important sexual parts and boost sexual performance.

• Chilies and peppers. All-natural spicy foods help your blood flow by reducing hypertension and inflammation.

3. Eat these meats and other foods

Here are some more foods that can help you achieve better blood flow:

• Omega-3 fatty acids. This type of fat increases blood flow. You can find it in salmon, tuna, avocados, and olive oil.

• Vitamin B-1. This vitamin helps signals in your nervous system move quicker, including signals from your brain to your penis. It's found in pork, peanuts, and kidney beans.

• Eggs. High in other B vitamins, eggs help balance hormone levels. This can decrease stress that often inhibits an erection.

4. Reduce stress

Stress can affect all areas of your health, including your libido.

Stress increases your heart rate (in the bad way) and increases blood pressure. Both of these are damaging to sexual desire and performance.

Psychological stress can also affect achieving an erection or reaching an orgasm.

Exercise is a great way to reduce stress and improve your health.

Talking to your partner about your stress can also calm you down, while strengthening your relationship at the same time.

Stress can also trigger bad habits, such as smoking or alcohol consumption, which can harm your sexual performance.

5. Kick bad habits

What you rely on to unwind, such as smoking and consuming alcohol, could also affect sexual performance.

While studies suggest that a little red wine can improve circulation, too much alcohol can have adverse effects.

Stimulants narrow blood vessels and have been linked to impotence. Cutting down or quitting smoking is one of the first steps to improve performance.

Replacing bad habits with healthy ones, such as exercise and eating well, can help boost sexual health.

6. Get some sun

Sunlight stops the body's production of melatonin. This hormone helps us sleep but also quiets our sexual urges. Less melatonin means the potential for more sexual desire.

Getting outside and letting the sun hit your skin can help wake up your sex drive, especially during the winter months when the body produces more melatonin.

7. Masturbate to improve longevity

If you're not lasting as long as you'd like in bed, you might need some practice. While sex is the best way to practice for sex, masturbation can also help you improve your longevity.

However, how you masturbate could have detrimental effects. If you rush through it, you could inadvertently decrease the time you last with your partner. The secret is making it last, just like you want to when you're not alone.

8. Pay attention to your partner

Sex isn't a one-way street. Paying special attention to your partner's desires not only makes sex pleasurable for them, but it can also help turn you on or slow you down. Talking about this beforehand can help ease any awkwardness if you need to slow down during a heated moment.

Alternating pace or focusing on your partner while you take a break can make for a more enjoyable experience for both of you.

9. Get more help if you need it

If you have erectile dysfunction, Peyronie's disease, or other diagnosed disorders, you may need medical treatment. Don't hesitate to talk to your doctor about how you can improve your sexual performance.

It's never a bad decision to exercise, eat right, and enjoy your sex life to the fullest.

9 Safe Ways to Increase Female Libido

Causes of low libido

Decreased libido in women can happen at any time after you've become sexually active. Most women experience it a lot after pregnancy when breastfeeding.

Also, your libido could go crashing from hundred back to zero due to anxiety, stress, or hormonal imbalance due to changes in the body. Even certain level of sexual disorders can cause loss of libido in women.

Whatever be the reason for your decreased libido, it shouldn't cause you more anxiety or be the reason you shy away from trying to get the green light on again for your partner. Why is that? Lowered libido isn't a sentence and there are different ways to increase it.

Solutions for low libido in women

Exercise more

Different home treatments and remedies exist, some of which you can whip up on your own to get your sexual drive up. One of

the reasons for lack of sex drive in females
might be lack of exercise. Exercise is needed
for an optimally healthy body and so your
doctor might suggest you add it to your list
of healthy things to help increase your
libido.

Exercising more than your daily walk to the
grocery store or to that park around the
corner is the best natural libido booster that
you can get for free. It might just cost you a
few drops of sweat though but what is that
compared to the joy that comes with having
your libido back.

Whatever exercise you have to do; be it
yoga or just running from one block to
another or possibly jogging about the park,
once it helps you connect more to your body
and be aware of yourself, you are one step to

skyrocketing that libido then. Most doctors suggest exercise as it would help you feel a lot more at ease and confident in the bedroom.

You know one exercise that gives you guts? Taking boxing class. You could try that as you might need all the guts and confidence you can get if you are having a case of lowered libido due to low self-esteem or mental health issues.

Certain pelvic exercises could also go a long way to help your muscles relax so if your doctor suggests Kegels to help your pelvic region as the muscles around there are responsible for contraction during orgasm, then follow her recommendations. You never know, it might be that missing piece you haven't tried yet.

Cope with stress

Learning to handle stress in a positive way can increase female sex drive. Rubbing your stress and anxiety in his face doesn't help him notice how stressed you are, it only gives him more stress more especially when he has been trying to get you aroused all to no avail. Get rid of your stress somehow.

Your doctor might suggest meditation. That's one of the best ways to cope with your stress. Whenever you are feeling your anxiety toping the charts, you can go into your room or whatever quiet place you've chosen, clear your head of all the troubling thoughts meditate on how beautiful life is and the fact that having your partner still craving for you is one of the best things ever. Look at stress as call to action as regards your lifestyle and make positive changes on yourself with it.

Once you've dealt with all the stress, your body will relax and you can have your libido back and intact.

Talk to your partner

Spending time and actually talking to your partner goes a long way to get you back in the game. Every woman, no matter how busy you get, should spend at least 20 minutes of talking time with her partner. This time should be just for your partner and not interrupted by social media or any electronics.

Communication can help him understand how to help you get your libido back. It would help him know if prolonged foreplay will do the trick for you or probably talking in a sensuous way to you. However it may be, set aside partner time and communicate.

Spice up your love life

Having just one particular prim and proper way to initiate sex every time could cause female libido problems. Sex becomes boring and you gradually lose interest. At this point, spicing up your love life by coming up with different other ways to arouse your spouse or teaching him different other ways to get you in the game could go a long way to tackle your decreased libido.

Get plenty of sleep

A hectic lifestyle can snatch your precious sleep from you and therefore making weary and stressed out. Sleep helps your nerves relax and in turn helps your body to function normally. When the body gets less sleep and more stressed out, you tend to lose interest in a lot of things. Exhaustion lowers your sex drive and so getting enough sleep or taking power naps when you can while accompanying it with rich-in-protein diet can go a long way in increasing your sex drive.

Sex drive foods

Eating a lot more chocolate might be that home remedy that works for you. You know what they say about chocolate and the fact that it symbolizes desire. This is not just because of its mind blowing taste that sets your taste buds on fire and longing for more once it comes in contact with them.

A study done on chocolate shows that it helps in the secretion of more serotonin in your body. Doctors all over the world say that this hormone is responsible for putting you in an aphrodisiac mood. Guess what it does to your body? It longs for a males touch after a dose of chocolates or some other pleasurable foods like figs, oysters or peaches. You could decide to combine the two famous aphrodisiacs: chocolate and oysters.

If eating these two gets you feeling sensuous or feels pleasurable, then get ready to be fired up for a long time action. Treating yourself to a homemade dish with these two as dessert might leave you wanting a lot more than dessert to quench the sensuous feeling it has awoken.

Eating a lot of fruits can be another great home treatment for a lowered sex drive in females. Some certain fruits have been found and suggested by doctors for consumption during this time of your life as a woman. Apart from the fruits already mentioned, other fruits such as bananas, and avocado not only boost your libido but also increases blood flow to the genitals and therefore promoting a normal and healthy sex life.

Make an appointment with your practitioner

Consulting your health practitioner for a case of decreased libido is one of the wisest things you should do before you embark on any form of treatment or therapy.

Whether or not you think the natural approach is the best for you, making an appointment with your health practitioner to let him or her know about your libido problems can go a long way to help you find out if your libido issue is just due to stress or some other underlying problems. Most times your libido could be as a result of female lubrication problems or some other underlying medical conditions which could be mental or otherwise.

Whatever the problem might be, your doctor will be the only one to let you know the root of the problem affecting your sex life. This makes it easier to find a solution to whatever sexual problem you are facing.

Medication

Different medications for the increase of female sex drive exist. Before you think of taking any libido enhancer for women, always ensure that you consult your doctor. He or she can tell you whether or not your body can handle these enhancers and which one to use. Some herbs which contain certain alkaloids or ingredients that boost your libido exist and can be used as a natural Viagra but before you go herbal or orthodox, involve your doctor.

Hormone treatment

Hormonal imbalance can be the cause of decreased libido in women and so in order to correct this, doctors place these women on a hormone treatment therapy in order to boost the different hormones involved in the inciting pleasure for a healthy and enjoyable sex. It is important to let your doctor suggest what sort of hormone treatment therapy you should be placed on.

What are sex pills?

Generally, 'sex pills' is the name people give to pills you take for a few specific sex-related problems or to improve the quality of their sex life in general.

'Sex pills' do include real medications that work and can be recommended by doctors. But, there are also pills that are unlicensed, herbal, or sold over-the-counter, which aren't proven to work, aren't properly checked to make sure they're safe.

If you don't have a specific sex-related problem and you're just looking to improve your sex life, sex pills probably aren't the right call.

Before thinking about what pill to try for your sex life, it's a good idea to think about what you want from your sex life and what might be the best and safest way to make it happen. Often, you can see big improvements to your sex life by making changes to your lifestyle, getting counselling or therapy, or talking things through with your partner.

What are the best sex pills available?

The best sex pills around are ones that are from a regulated service that includes qualified doctors or pharmacists. This includes medications for premature ejaculation (PE) and erectile dysfunction (ED):

• ED pills – Viagra (sildenafil) and other pills like Viagra

• PE pills – Priligy (dapoxetine)

If you don't have ED or PE, or if the medications available for PE or ED aren't safe or effective for you, then unfortunately there aren't any better alternative pills. If these treatments aren't safe for you, you can either try non-pill medications, like EMLA for PE, or a vacuum pump for ED, or else you could try non-medical treatments like counselling, lifestyle changes, surgery, or others.

Understandably, you might want a herbal pill that you can get hold of without having to get assessed first. The reality is though, that there's no 'best sex pill' because none of them are proven to work. Even though it's not ideal, treating sex-related problems or improving your sex life might mean looking at solutions other than a pill.

What are erection pills?

People usually think of 2 different outcomes when they talk about erection pills:

• Pills used to treat erectile dysfunction (ED)

• Pills marketed at improving your maximum erection size, which don't actually work

Treating ED

• ED pills can help you if you can't reach or stay at your natural maximum erection size, but they won't increase your maximum erection size

• You can find ED pills that are real medications which work, but you can also find herbal ED pills too

• You can order real ED medication online, from a pharmacist, or from your GP, as long as you have ED and the pills are safe for you

Improving your erection size

There aren't any pill that can really improve your maximum erection size. You shouldn't go in for any products that make this claim, because they won't work and they might not be safe. The only way to increase your maximum erection size is through surgery.

What are male enhancement pills?

Generally speaking, 'male enhancement pills' describe pills marketed to men that have mixtures of different herbal ingredients, and sellers often claim they will improve sexual performance and/or increase penis size.

There's no medical proof that these kinds of pills do what they claim to, so you might want to think twice about buying and using them. If you do decide to use these kinds of pills, at least make sure the seller is the real deal and check that the pills have been approved by the right organisations. Ideally, you also want to talk to your doctor first before trying these kinds of products.

Are male enhancement pills dangerous?

Possible side effects:

• Normally, medications are carefully
checked – it's clear what the ingredients are
and how much of them there is, and this
helps professionals decide whether it's safe
or not

• Male enhancement pills aren't checked in
the same way, if at all

• So, we don't know if they really contain
what they say they do

• Even if the ingredients are correct, in the
amounts that the seller says, and the
ingredients on their own are safe, they might
not be safe mixed together

• Because of the points above, it's hard to
tell what side effects male enhancement pills
could cause, or how serious they might be

• If male enhancement pills do have any medical effects, or if they actually have some actually medications mixed in, then there could be a risk of serious side effects

Taking unnecessary risks:

• Apart from possible side effects, the biggest downside to buying male enhancement pills is that they probably won't work

• Only proper medications are proven to help safely sex-related problems

• If you try male enhancement products like these, you're putting yourself at risk of the side effects, without getting any benefits in return

• Even if these pills aren't dangerous, you could still be paying out money for nothing

• Claims that these kinds of products work isn't based on proper scientific evidence, like real medications – at best, there might be one or two small studies that show some benefits, but that's not enough to prove anything

• So, none of these male enhancement products would ever be recommended for you by a doctor or pharmacist

Are there sex pills for women?

Women can also get sex-related problems, like:

• Low sex drive

• Feeling pain during sex

• Having problems getting an orgasm

There's currently no medication available in the UK specifically for treating sexual problems in women. But there are some medications that might work, that are available in other countries. Still there's not enough proof for them to be sold in the UK.

Flibanserin

This medication is available in the US for low sex drive in women who haven't gone through menopause. It's been licenced since 2015, but it can't be used for all the causes of low sex drive, like when it's caused by different medical conditions or relationship problems. There are mixed reviews on Flibanserin, so it's hard to tell if this could help improve your sex drive or not. Either way, it's not available in the UK.

Selective serotonin reuptake inhibitors (SSRIs)

These are drugs that you'd usually be prescribed if you had depression or anxiety, but they can also be used for premature ejaculation in men. These medications might be able to help if you sex problems are being caused by a mental health problem like depression or anxiety. On the other hand, SSRIs can also cause low sex drive and stop you from being able to orgasm as side effects.

Prelox

This is a herbal product marketed at improving sex problems in women who've been through the menopause. It contains ingredients that are thought to improve sexual problems in women, but there's a lot of mixed information on whether they work. Like with male enhancement products, using herbal products like Prelox isn't a good idea.

Sex therapy or counselling

Your thoughts and feelings can have a big impact on lots of aspects of your life, including your sex life. Talking to a sex therapist or counsellor could help you explore your problems and help deal with some of the roots causes.

Just like with men, a lot of factors can affect you sex life, like physical problems, mental health problems, or relationship problems. Talking to a doctor or therapist could help you suss out where your problems are coming from and what steps to take to start improving them.

Are there pills to help you last longer in bed?

The medications that'll help you last longer in bed will depend on why you normally have to stop having sex sooner than you want to.

Pills to make your erections last longer

If you can't get or keep your erections and that's why you can't last longer in bed, there are treatments available. Some of the licensed treatments for erection problems include Viagra, Sildenafil, Levitra, and Cialis.

Pill to stop you ejaculating as quickly

If you can't last longer in bed because you're coming too quickly, there are also medications available. Examples include antidepressants (like Lexapro, Paxil, or Priligy), or painkillers (like Ultram).

Pills to stop you getting tired in bed

If you have to stop having sex because you're too tired there aren't any others pills you can safely take to stop you getting tired in the bedroom. The best thing to do is to improve your physical fitness overall.

Other things you can do to improve the sex you're having

There are a few different lifestyle changes, treatments, techniques and so on, which can have a positive impact on your sex life, including:

• Topical treatments for premature
ejaculation or erectile dysfunction – EMLA
or alprostadil

• Techniques for premature ejaculation – the
'start-stop' technique, the 'squeeze'
technique

• Penis pumps or rings for erectile
dysfunction

• Pelvic floor exercises

• Maintaining a healthy diet and weight

• Getting enough general exercise

• Counselling or therapy

• Getting a medications review to see if any
of your current meds are causing your
sexual problems

• Checking for underlying health conditions – diabetes, thyroid problems etc, that might be causing your problems

Factors affecting sexual desire

Levels of sexual desire may fluctuate over time due to internal and external factors.

Social and relationship influences

One's social situation can refer to the social circumstances of life, the stage of life one is in, the state of one's relationship with a partner, or even if there is a relationship at all. Whether people think that their experience of desire or lack of experience is problematic depends on special kinds of social circumstances such as the presence or absence of a partner.[6][8] As social beings, many humans seek out lifetime partners and wish to experience that celebrated connection and intimacy. Sexual desire is often considered essential to romantic attraction and relationship development.[1] The experience of desire can ebb and flow with the passing of time, with increasing familiarity for one's partner, and with the changing of relationship dynamics and priorities..

Disorders

There are currently two Sexual Desire
Disorders in the Diagnostic and Statistical
Manual IV-TR (DSM-IV-TR) which affect
men and women alike. The first is
hypoactive sexual desire disorder (HSDD).
HSDD is currently defined by the DSM as
"persistently or recurrently deficient (or
absent) sexual fantasies and desire for sexual
activity" which causes "marked distress or
interpersonal difficulty". However, this
definition has been met with some
disagreement in recent years as it places too
much emphasis on Sexual Fantasy which are
usually used to supplement sexual arousal.
As a result, a group of sexuality researchers
and clinicians have recently proposed the
addition of Sexual Desire/Interest Disorder
(SDID) to the DSM in hopes that it may

encompass sexual desire concerns specifically in women more accurately. SDID is defined by low sexual desire, absent sexual fantasies, and a lack of responsive desire.

The second Sexual Desire Disorder in the DSM is Sexual Aversion Disorder (SAD). SAD is defined as "persistent or recurrent extreme aversion to, and avoidance of, all or almost all, genital sexual contact with a sexual partner" However, some have questioned the placement of SAD within the sexual dysfunction category of the DSM and have called for its placement within the Specific phobia grouping as an Anxiety Disorder. Both HSDD and SAD has been found to be more prevalent in females than males, this is especially the case in SAD. However, on a spectrum of severity, HSDD would be considered less severe than SAD.

On the opposite end of the Sexual Desire Disorder spectrum is Hypersexual disorder. According to the proposed revision to the DSM which will include Hypersexual Disorder in the appendix of future publications, Hypersexual Disorder is defined as "recurrent and intense sexual fantasies, sexual urges, and sexual behavior" where the individual is consumed with excessive sexual desire and repeatedly engages in sexual behavior in response to "dysphoric mood states and stressful life events". Hypersexual Disorder is currently associated with sexual addiction and sexual compulsivity.

Health

A serious or chronic illness can have an enormous effect on the biological drive and the psychological motivation for sexual desire and sexual behaviour. With poor health, an individual may be able to experience some desire but does not have the motivation or strength to have sex. Physical and mental well-being is crucial to successful and satisfying sexual expression. Chronic disorders like cardiovascular disease, diabetes, arthritis, enlarged prostates (in men), Parkinson's disease, and cancer can have negative influence over sexual desire, sexual functioning, and sexual response. In the case of diabetes, especially in men, there have been conflicting findings of the effect of the disease on sexual desire. Some studies have found that diabetic men have shown lower levels of sexual desire than healthy, age-matched counterparts. While other researchers have found no difference in level of sexual desire between diabetic men and healthy controls. High-blood pressure has also been found to be related to declining levels of sexual desire in men and women alike.

Medications

Certain medications can cause changes in the level of experienced sexual desire through "non-specific effects on general well-being, energy level, and mood".

Declining levels of sexual desire have been linked to the use of anti-hypertension medication and many psychiatric medications; such as anti-psychotic medications, tricyclic anti-depressants, monoamine-oxidase (MAO) inhibitors, and sedative drugs. However, the most severe decreases in sexual desire relating to psychiatric medication occur due to the use of selective serotonin reuptake inhibitors (SSRIs). In women specifically, the use of anticoagulants, cardiovascular medications, medications to control cholesterol, and medications for hypertension contributed to low levels of desire. However, in men, only the use of anticoagulants and medications for hypertension was related to low levels of desire. In addition to the specific type of medication being used, the amount of medications used regularly was also found to be correlated with a lowering of sexual desire. One medication that many do not realize can lower sexual desire in women is the oral contraceptive. Not every woman experiences the negative side effects of the pill, however, as many as one in four do. In addition, the pill reduces the sexual attractiveness of women by changing their estrus phase.[36] Oral contraceptives have been known to increase the levels of sex hormone-binding globulin (SHBG) in the body. In turn, high SHBG levels have been associated with a decline in sexual desire. Though it is not used as medication, the drug methamphetamine has a strong positive effect on many aspects of sexual behaviour, including sexual desire.

Hormones

Sexual desire is said to be influenced by androgens in men and by androgens and estrogens in women. Many studies associate the sex hormone, testosterone with sexual desire. Testosterone is mainly synthesized in the testes in men and in the ovaries in women. Another hormone thought to influence sexual desire is oxytocin. Exogenous administration of moderate amounts of oxytocin has been found to stimulate females to desire and seek out sexual activity.[9] In women, oxytocin levels are at their highest during sexual activity. In males, the frequency of ejaculations affects the libido. If the gap between ejaculations extends toward a week, there will be a stronger desire for sexual activity.

Interventions

There are a few medical interventions that can be done on individuals who feel sexually bored, experience performance anxiety, or are unable to orgasm. For everyday life, a 2013 fact sheet by the Association for Reproductive Health Professionals recommends:

Erotic literature

Recalling instances when felt sexy and sexual ("The patient is instructed to recall her physical appearance, the setting, the smells in the air, the music she was hearing, and the foods she was eating at that time and use these as 'cues' for feeling sexual now")

www.ingramcontent.com/pod-product-compliance
Lightning Source LLC
Chambersburg PA
CBHW022228160726
47991CB00016B/2652